Table of Contents

CHAPTER 1
Get Yourself Ready

Introduction

I can't believe I'm actually penning the book that will enable you to attain the level of fitness and health of which you have only ever dreamed. Me, who could barely run a block in gym class and was always last picked. A good story has power, so here is mine:

Most of my upbringing and early adulthood were dominated by health issues. Since I can remember, I have struggled with terrible allergies, asthma, a spastic colon, irritable bowel syndrome, and low self-esteem. I was ill, frail, and defeated as a child. I was advised to take it easy, take my medications on schedule, and try to make the best of it.

Sports were obviously out because I wasn't allowed to play outside for fear of my allergies and asthma "getting stirred up." I tried playing softball one year, but it's hard to want to try anything if you frequently get made fun of, so I didn't play much. Due to my spastic colon, illness, and poor diet, I spent a lot of time in the emergency department throughout my college years for "tummy" issues. I struggled with my health right up until I was in my mid-20s. I eventually grew Sick And Tired of feeling that way. I had to regain initiative and reclaim my life.

I concentrated on food and what it meant for my body. I started to pursue better decisions and was passed up the manner in which I began to feel. I had energy, felt perfect and best of all my illness and "belly issues" recently vanished! I felt so great that I began to work out. Me, exercise! Amazing! It was difficult and I needed to creep before I could walk But I Did It! This fellow who lacked the ability to run in exercise center class or do a solitary push up was running everyday and lifting loads. I was unable to accept how my body was changing before my eyes. What flabbergasted me the most was that my sensitivities even improved, any who body experiences them knows how huge of an explanation that is! I assumed command over my wellbeing which in the long run assisted me with zeroing in more on my marriage (almost 15 years and more grounded than at any other time), plunge further in my confidence, gain self-assurance and arrive at a level satisfaction in life I never imagined.

I'm sensitivity, asthma, spastic colon and ill-free. I at long last found harmony in my own body (internally and externally) and I am looking great. I currently invest wholeheartedly in committing my opportunity to helping other people feel improved and look over and above anyone's expectations previously.

So would you say you are prepared for this sort of life change? Is it true that you are weary of being heavy and dull?

It's fine.... there's hope!

"Without Determination Change is Unrealistic"

(Godwin Mathew)

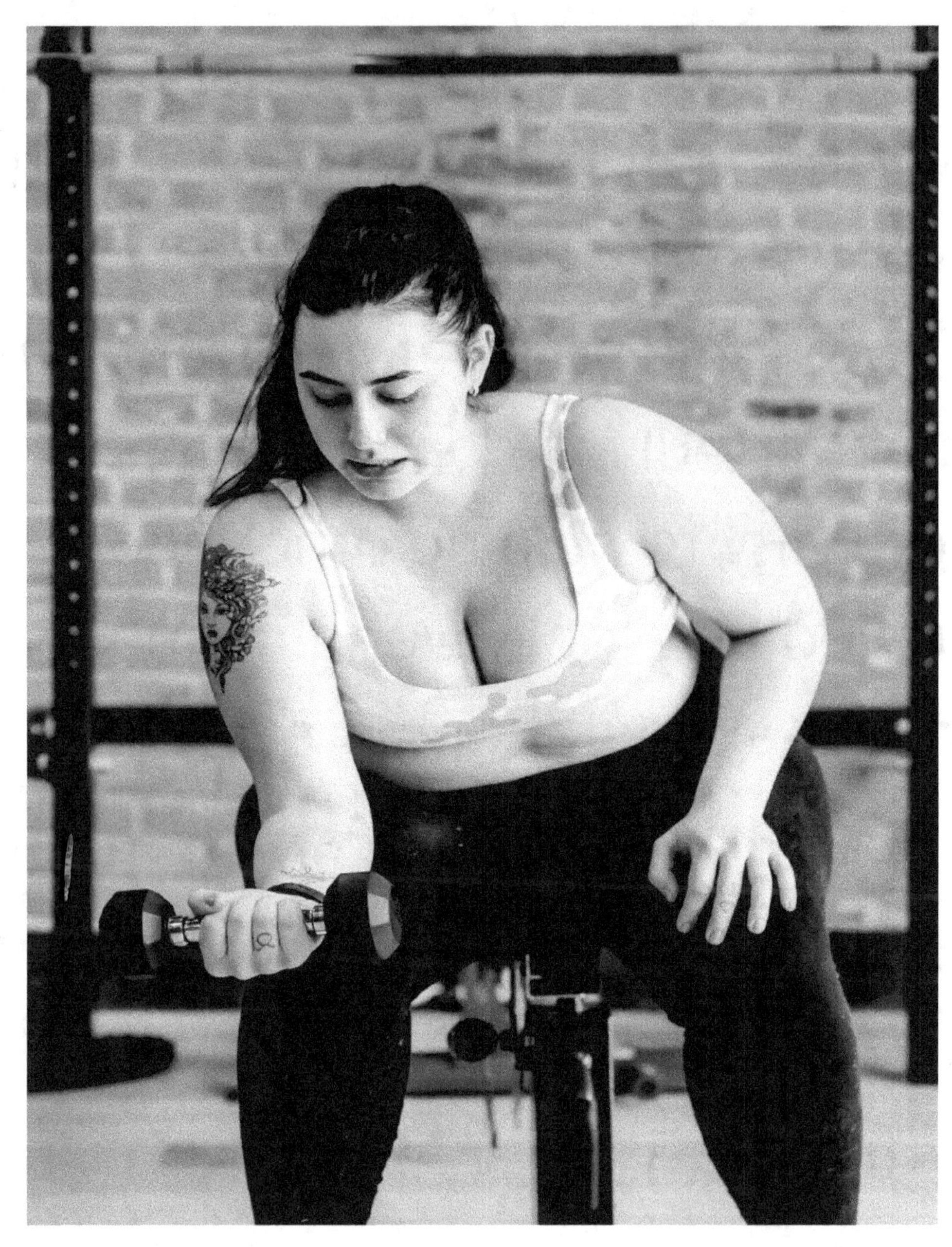

The Journey So Far

I have prepared many individuals

throughout the long term. I have prepared the youthful, old, over-weight, under-weight, athletic and stationary. There is one key component they should have before I will try and start to prepare them- they should be prepared to change their way of life.

You should make changes to your dietary patterns and exercise consistently.

You should scale back specific food varieties and carve out opportunity in your bustling timetable for work out. It will amaze you the number of individuals that anticipate significant change for almost no work. You have to learn not to depend on Weight Loss pill items because they don't really work more often than not.

I don't do calories counts. I request that individuals stop the handy solution mindset and begin putting resources into super durable way of life change. Ooohhhhh, I know that sounds so unnerving at present however I'm not looking at surrendering chocolate cake and pizza until the end of your life. I'm discussing control and all the more critically - BALANCE.

So you really want to seriously investigate your life, responsibility level and the significance of this adjustment of your life.

Is it safe to say that you are prepared?

 Begin with the KIS plan...

(Keep It Simple)

Being sound isn't super complicated;

=> Teach yourself so there is no doubt as far as you can tell about how you ought to work out furthermore, what you ought to eat.

=> Encircle yourself with individuals, spots and things that will support your advancement.

=> Don't overanalyze everything... JUST DO IT! Without a doubt, you will mess up however you will learn from those missteps.

"Yet, I have attempted and failed so often previously." Let me ask you... was it a reasonable, sound program? Or on the other hand was it a convenient solution in a jug, no carbs, no fat, stand on your head and essentially make-you-hopeless program?

Diet programs that make ridiculous cases and request you to kill key components from a reasonable eating routine DO NOT WORK!

The watchword is BALANCE!

"Success is not Cheap Even Though it's Affordable."

(Godwin Mathew)

My program is very easy to follow...

FITNESS + NUTRITION + MOTIVATION = WEIGHT LOSS SUCCESS

This is what I will like you to do:

Conceive It

Know your objectives. You should know why you need to make changes and all the more significantly ARE YOU READY FOR CHANGE. Large number of us need to shed pounds and become fit yet when it comes down to it, we would rather not accomplish the work or change our way of life. You should have a prepared brain and open heart before any sure changes can happen. We will discuss these regions later.

Believe It

Accept you can make it happen! Regardless of how frequently you have begun new "diets" and "crazy exercises" realize that you can change. You are the main thing preventing you from Victory. You should accept that ideal wellbeing is inside your scope.

Achieve It

Don't mind the cost, just do how you realize you want to help your actual wellbeing yet in addition for your psychological and otherwise wellbeing. By accomplishing better wellbeing you reward yourself with more energy, fearlessness, better mentality and an engaged soul.

There is no restriction to what you can accomplish.

What Should be Your Motivation?

>> What is in our future in the event that we don't make progress with our unfortunate things to do?

>> Don't we owe it to our family?

  We should require a moment to do a truly educational activity:

>> Push ahead to when your kids (kid) are developed. Assuming that you do not have youngsters utilize another relative or companion. I maintain that you should compose

their account as though you passed on today. What will your kid's (or other) life be like? What will it mean for them assuming you keep on the way that you are on right presently?

>> Presently compose the history as though you roll out the improvements you realize you want to make. How might their life be impacted assuming you settle on better decisions and way of life changes today.

Amazing, enlightening stuff right? Let's move ahead......

Where Do You Start?

>> What are your (reasonable) present moment, long haul and persuasive objectives?

>> Make an arrangement utilizing a day to day log book.

>> Picture your breakthrough!

>> Ponder/Pray for support at snapshots of shortcoming and to recover pivot.

>> Teach yourself on what and how you want to eat and work out.

How Do You Take Action?

>> Try not to count calories! Make solid way of life changes. Individuals don't fall flat at eating less, abstains from food affect individuals!

>> Find what practice you like and focus on it! No more reasons to quit.

>> Teach yourself on how, what and when to eat refreshingly.

>> Find somebody who will support you, develop you and be uncompromising with you (in a

caring way). You really want somebody to consider you responsible!

Enlist a mentor or inquire a companion... don't act like a lone cruiser.

Do You Consider Yourself Set......Then Let's Gooo...

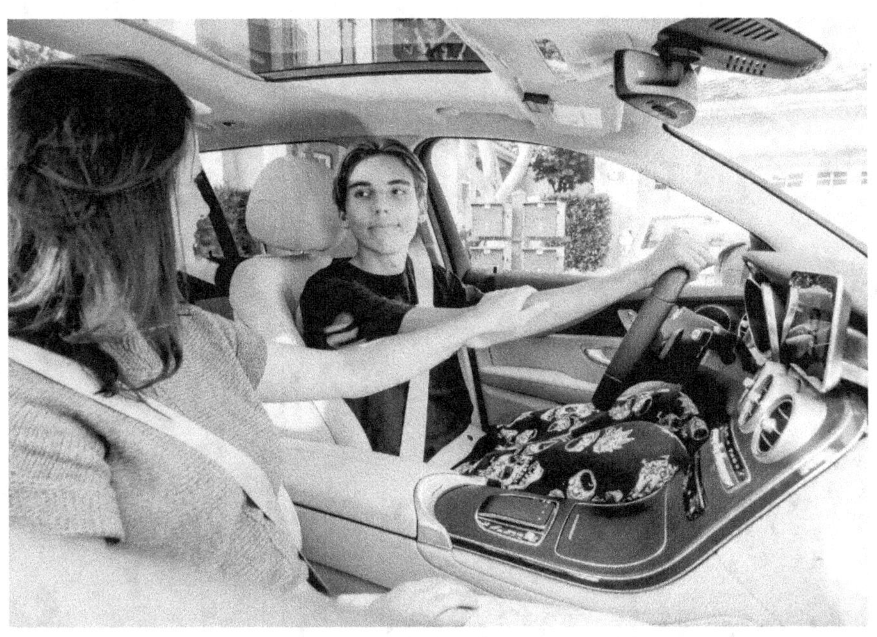

CHAPTER 2
Discard Poor Diet Thought Pattern

Before you could actually ponder what to eat and how to exercise you really want to get into your head. I have watched a lot of individuals start the way of life change process just to stop three or four weeks after the fact. There is something else to it than eating right and working out. You MUST dig somewhere inside to figure out what drove to your ongoing wellbeing status and figure out what will persuade you to victory.

Let's unwrap the pack further.....

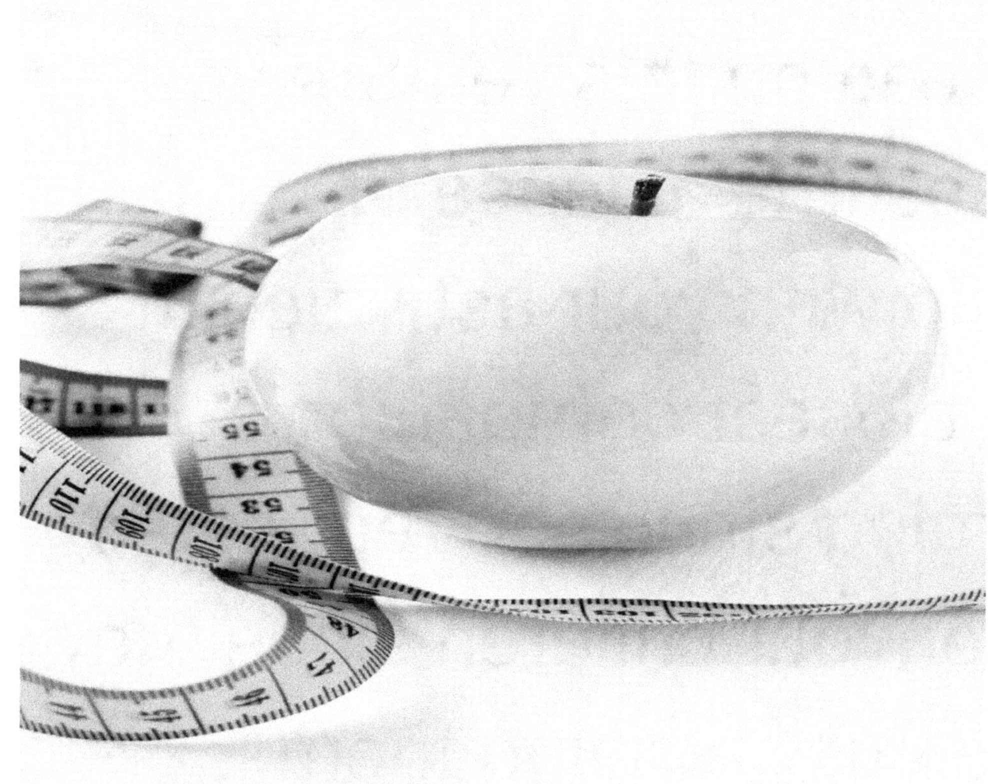

TAKE RESPONSIBILITY

You found yourself mixed up with

this wreck currently it depends on you to get yourself out! Nobody constrained you to put on weight or become unfortunate. Before you can proceed on this venture you should assume a sense of ownership with your activities. It's not your closest companion's shortcoming since she requested dessert or your children since they keep you busy running them around. You go with your own decisions and the sooner you understand the ball is continuously in your court the nearer you are to weight reduction achievement.

LET THE PAST GO

No doubt, you've pursued a few unfortunate decisions before. That multitude of decisions have driven you

to the shape you're in the present moment. For what reason do we eat a whole box of Candy Chocolate treats all at once? For what reason truly do we involve our treadmill as a garments line? There are quite a large number of purposes behind this way of behaving: self indulgence, unfortunate demeanor, misery, absence of concentration, no plan, lethargy, no resolve, personal strife and stress, to give some examples. Some times there can be profound personal scars from a youth injury or close to home occasion that should be tended to. Once in a while these sort of repressed feelings can forestall weight reduction or way of life change. I prescribe seeing a specialist or minister to really focus on the main thing. Abandon all that old stuff and begin clean. The enhanced you is not far off.

PUT A CHECK ON YOUR ATTITUDE

Another key component that could decide whether you are effective in changing your way of life is YOUR ATTITUDE. Individuals who have an uplifting outlook are in every case more effective in weight reduction too. They let their "I can't" necessities to change to "I will". Self attestation is extremely strong.

Negative reasoning brings up self question, dread and discontent. It is the very fuel that makes and supports a negative inward climate. Basically:

Change your thinking and your body will follow!

Please Consider this Task: Make a rundown of certain things you will acquire from exercise and eating better. Post this rundown on the washroom mirror, refrigerator or in your vehicle, that way you will be continually helped to remember what you need to acquire by staying with your new solid way of life.

AVOID EMOTIONAL EATING

One of the greatest adversaries of weight reduction is Emotional Eating. That may sound funny, this is associated with eating carelessly just because you are exhausted, pushed, had a battle with somebody, and so on. The vast majority of us have done this sooner or later in our lives however when it occurs consistently it is a MAJOR issue. You want to figure out how to deal with these snapshots of shortcoming with positive other options from there, the sky is the limit, critically figure out how to head them off before they occur. Understanding what sets off these occasions will turn out to be vital in your general achievement.

DUMP ALL UNREALISTIC

EXPECTATIONS (BE REAL)

Every one of your concerns won't be addressed in the event that you shed some pounds of fat.

In any case, the excursion to arrive may simply completely change you. Each move toward your excursion to better wellbeing will show you your assets, shortcomings, instruct you about appropriate sustenance and exercise as well as construct your self-certainty.

This is an excursion and your weight reduction and individual objectives are not going to be accomplished over night. It took a significant stretch of time to put the load on and IT WILL take a while to get it off too. You can go out and do a hardship, no carb, weight reduction in-a-jug or lack of hydration plan and lose a lot of water weight in seven days. Issue is you will feel like poop and restore it (to say the least) as quick as possible.

Listen people, you must do things another way than previously. You must put your time and centered energy into this thing.

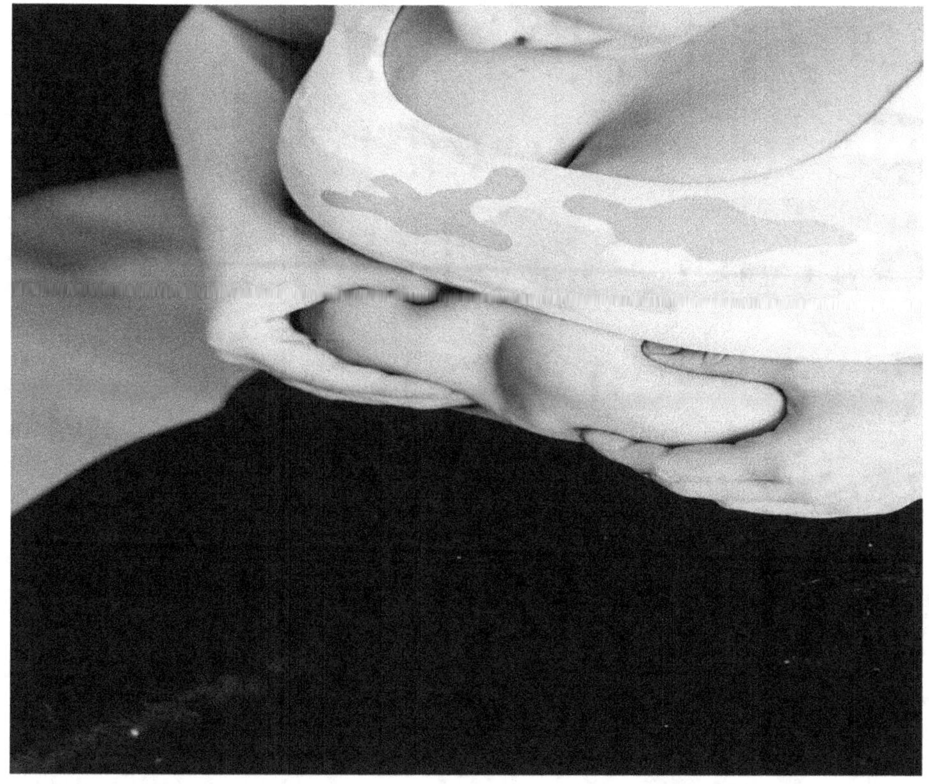

PUTTING THE WEIGHT OFF

A great many people believe that once they lose the weight they can return to carrying on with life as previously. Wouldn't you say that assuming you quit practicing and eating refreshingly your body couldn't pay heed? Wow! The devices, abilities and way of life you are going to learn are guardians. In the event that you return to your prior ways, I GUARANTEE you will recapture each pounds of fat (to say the least) you endeavored to lose. In all actuality the new you won't need the old way of life back. You will acquire so many great things by further developing your wellbeing that I question you will at any point return to your prior ways.

Know about triggers:

=>The young lady in the workplace who is continuously bringing you heated merchandise.

=>Your "dearest companion" who pushes you to flounder in cheap food wretchedness with her.

=>Your over soothing guardian or

companion who needs to take care of the issues out of your life.

Anticipate these temptations coming and learn how to discipline yourself enough to avoid them.

ACCEPT THE NEW YOU

You have rolled out numerous improvements to get yourself where you are presently. You might be lighter, more invigorated, more spurred and more joyful than any time in recent memory. Embrace this new you. This excursion might have shown you qualities in your character that you never realized you had. Forge ahead with your process by including loved ones.

Together you can attempt new exercises and recipes. Show them how far you've come and rouse them to make a sound way of life of their own.

Utilize your freshly discovered energy and fearlessness to acquire another companion, view as a new love or set the sparkles back into and old one.

Thank goodness you look better now.... congratulations!

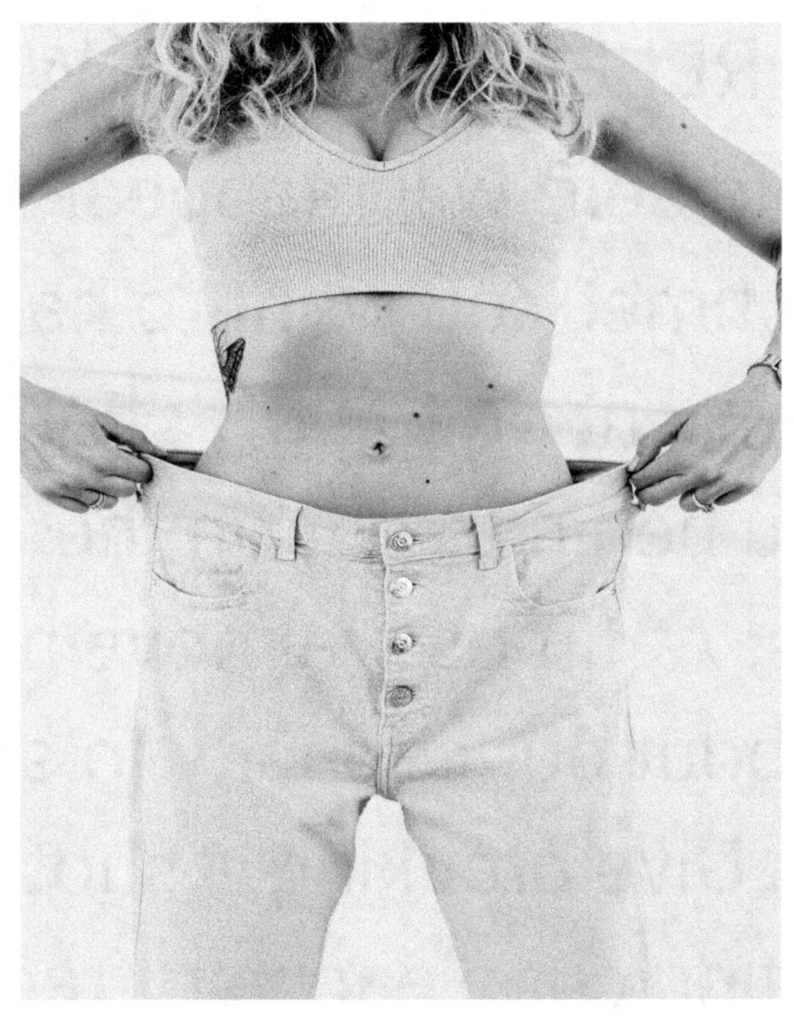

DON'T RELENT! KEEP A WATCH!

Your "old self" will reappear from time to time. You want to have an arrangement on the off chance that you begin to put on the pounds. At times we move past sure about our capacity to self-screen. Give breaking a shot the estimating cups each so frequently and really taking a look at your bits as opposed to eyeballing everything. Get out the venture diary and screen your eating so that seven days might check whether your eating is as "clean" as you suspect. Fruitful washouts keep it off when they know about their decisions and consistently in charge.

Rather than letting yourself know you "can't" have either food, take a stab at tracking down an approach to infrequently work it into your ongoing arrangement. I frequently add an additional walk or exercise type . I consume off the additional calories and hold my psychological mentality under tight restraints. In the event that I didn't do this I'm sure I would pound myself for a really long time and perhaps slip into another lavish expenditure meeting.

Think ahead and you can save yourself from long periods of disappointment.

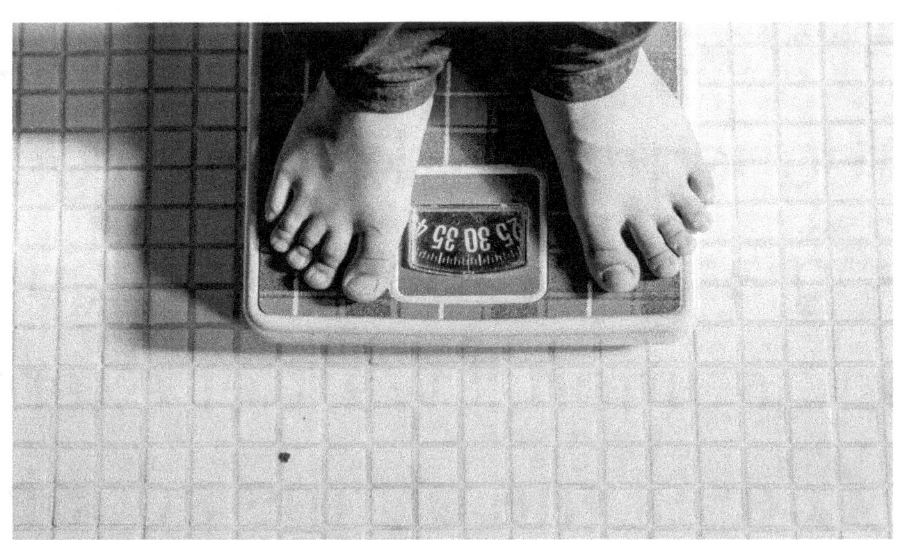

ENJOY YOUR NEW SYSTEM

Yeah...You did it! Always appreciate it! Ordinarily I see clients arrive at their weight reduction objectives just to be hopeless in light of the fact that they anticipated that their lives should do a 290 ° essentially on the grounds that they shed pounds. It isn't the scale numbers going down that gives joy it's the process and what you realized from it. It's great that you shed pounds yet more significantly you have found out about solid options, diving

profound into your fearlessness
and resolution.

CHAPTER 3

Build Your System On Right Facts

On the off chance that you simply hop in and fabricate your program without arranging it out you will once more wash away in the floods of dissatisfaction and disappointment. Assuming you set aside some margin to define objectives, plan your feasts, practice accurately and screen your advancement you will stand firm on that stone of achievement.

So how are you expected to build?

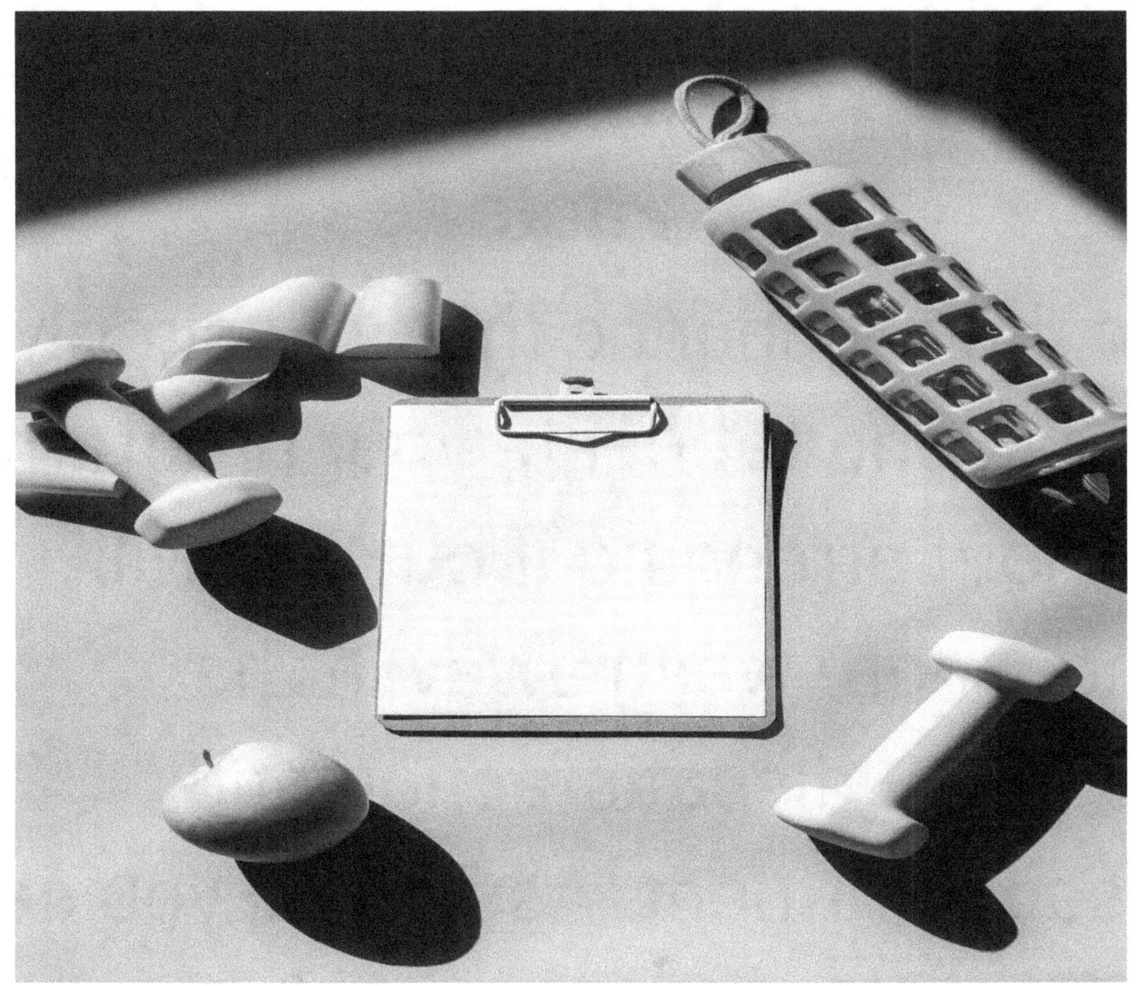

You Need To Set GOALS

Your weight loss goals should not be haphazard, it should be calculated and S.M.A.R.T(Specific, Measurable, Achievable, Realistic and Timely).

Getting more fit can be important for your general objective however you additionally need to have little momentary objectives, as well as, explicit, quantifiable long haul objectives. One of the key things you want to do while defining objectives isn't to incorporate "attempt". It isn't I will "attempt" to walk multiple times this week. It would be ideal for it to be...I "will" walk multiple times this week and I am focused on doing as such. You should be resolved to change and "attempt" isn't being dedicated. Saying you "will" do what you must to get it going, not allowing anything to hinder you.

What Short Term Goals Are: We should discuss transient objectives, these are the everyday or week by week objectives that are critical to your general achievement. They should be S.M.A.R.T. what's more, you really want to record them on paper and post them in a spot you will be continually reminded of what your central goal is. I suggest on the cooler entryway or washroom reflect.

Some Examples Are....

Week1:

I will walk multiple times this week and drink a full glass of water with each dinner.

Week2:

Go on with last weeks objectives, restrict myself to 1 inexpensive food dinner this week, supplant all sodas with water.

....

I think you understand. Every week you ought to roll out a sound improvement. In a little while you will have weaned off the prior ways and be headed to a less fatty, better you. In the event that you neglect to arrive at an objective, keep that equivalent objective the following week until the new sound propensity is set up.

What Long Term Goals Are:

Long haul objectives are similarly pretty much as significant as transient objectives. Long haul objectives are the 10,000 foot view and maintain the general focal point of your central goal. It is extremely, significant not to get yourself positioned for disappointment by defining unreasonable objectives. You shouldn't put forth a weight reduction objective of 50 pounds in two months. Assuming you drop that sort of quick weight reduction is risky and won't be long-lasting. Plus, on the event that you meet your objective sooner than anticipated you can simply make a new objective to keep you persuaded.

Some Examples Could Be:

=>I will lower my body fat by___%

=>I will lower my body pressure by___%

=>I will lower my body cholesterol by___% etc...

Motivational Goals Are Also Helpful:

You ought to likewise define

persuasive objectives. These objectives are substantially less ambiguous however and are similarly just about as significant as short and long haul objectives. These are the things that aren't quantifiable to anybody, yet you are the profound explanations behind your craving for way of life change. Picture your success!

Some Examples Are.....

=> I need to be the first in my family to break the weight cycle.

=> I need to acquire self-assurance.

=> I need to live agony free.

=> I would rather not be humiliated of my appearance any longer.

=>I need to have the option to demonstrate to everybody that I can change.

And when you reach your goals, learn to set new ones... good luck!

NEXT.....A JOURNEY JOURNAL

This is a truly significant device in your way of life change process. This is something beyond a food log, it is the means by which you will comprehend and perceive the occasions, individuals and circumstances that damage your achievement. Consider it... around early afternoon you had a major lunch (giant salad and other mixes) with your associate. At first you might think "a plate of mixed greens is sound" and "espresso isn't all that terrible and it's just a mix". At the point when you log this feast in your Journey Journal you find that the serving of mixed greens wound up having a greater number of calories and fat than a Big Mac and fries.

The Journey Journal permits you to see what season of day your "blow-it minutes" occurred and assists you with perceiving unfortunate examples in your eating routine.

Your Journey Journal Needs to Have the Following:

=> The date, day of the week,

=> Food and amount ate,

=> Season of feast and who you ate with,

=> Tow you felt when eating,

=> Absolute calories, protein, carbs and fat (discretionary),

=> Practice type, length, etc.

So basically you're documenting your behavior, intake and expenses. Other details are secondary.

OBSERVE YOUR PROGRESS RATE

Individuals learn in various ways: by contact, sight, hearing and doing. It's the same way while realizing what attempts to propel you. Some like to pay attention to persuading sound tapes while working out, others like to take bunch practice classes so they are encircled by individuals very much like them who have comparable objectives. Others need to see pictures that help them to remember where they need to be truly and that spur them to arrive at their objectives.

Always do things, go to places and surround yourself with people of like minds that will spur you to take your Weight Loss Tasks very seriously and be better at what you do.

Huge Success...

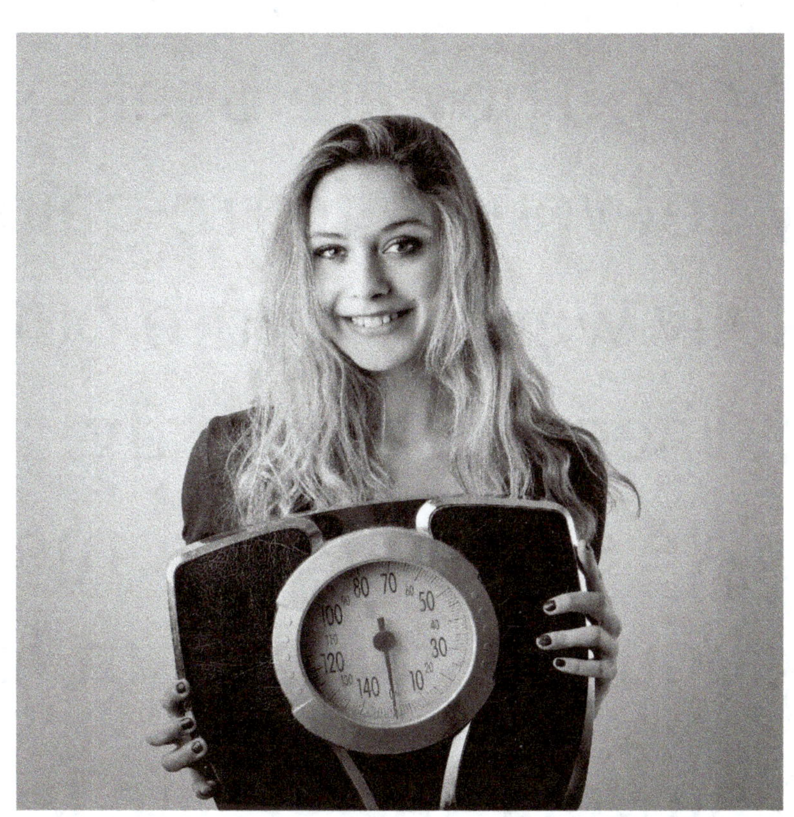

CHAPTER 4

The Need for Healthy Eating

For what reason do you assume you haven't kept the load off? Listen...counting calories/dieting don't work. They are brief sets that mainly set you up for re-gain later. You really want to figure out how to eat, when to eat and the amount to eat. We should talk somewhat more about abstains from food.

Changing your way of life is something worth being thankful for and doesn't include languishing.

Figure out how to settle on fortifying day to day decisions and exercise routinely and you can have it both ways!

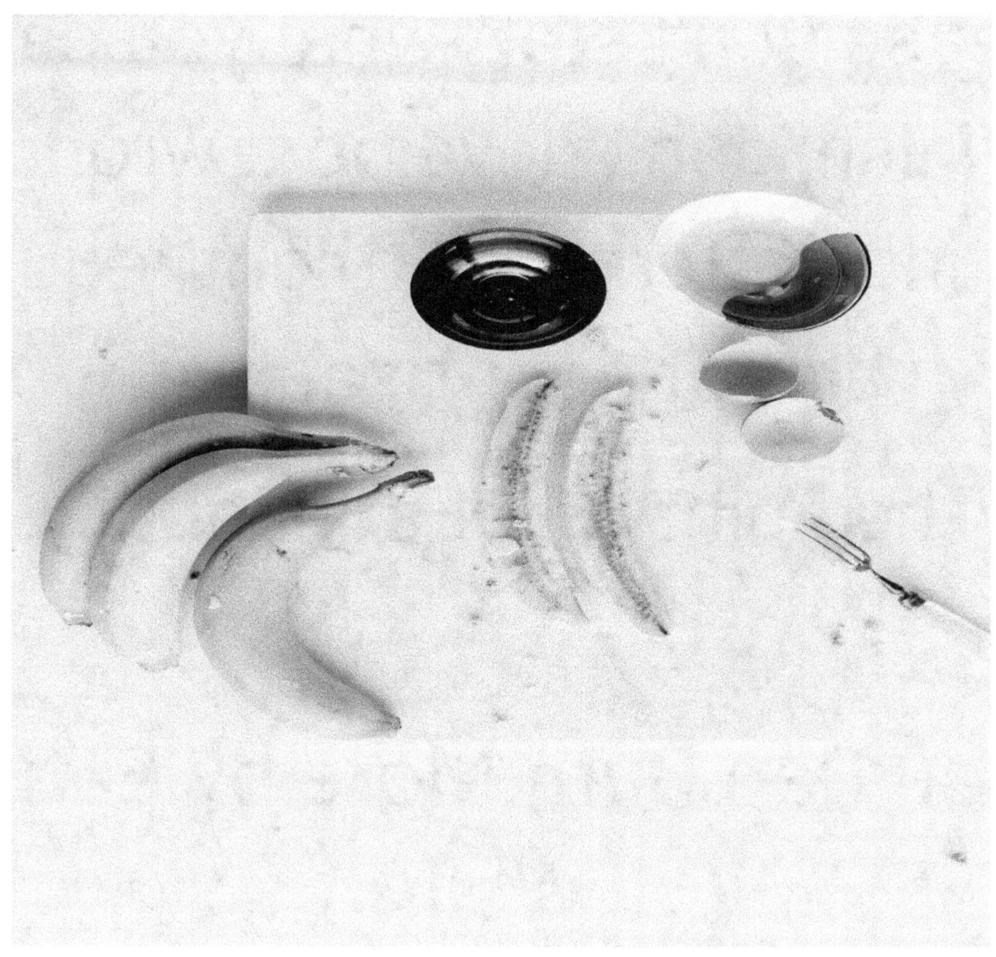

You are genuinely wasting your

experience with the handy solution, weight reduction in a jug, just protein, no eating, shed pounds in 24 hours joke programs, etc. But.... please don't start what you can't finish; don't develop a wrong eating pattern that might require alot of rigor to adjust.

The point is.....Eat healthily.

You Can Burn More by Eating Well

Indeed, exercises will assist you with consuming fat and calories yet how about we center around how to eat to consume. Little dinners on a more regular basis. Move away from the 2-3 huge feasts consistently. You ought to be training your body to be a consuming machine yet eating more modest feasts more often. Consider it... the vast majority skip breakfast and slow their digestion to a creep, then have a major lunch (frequently over eating since they are so starved), hit rock-bottom toward the middle of the day and have a soft drink jolt of energy and

return home to eat a major pasta
dinner with the family.

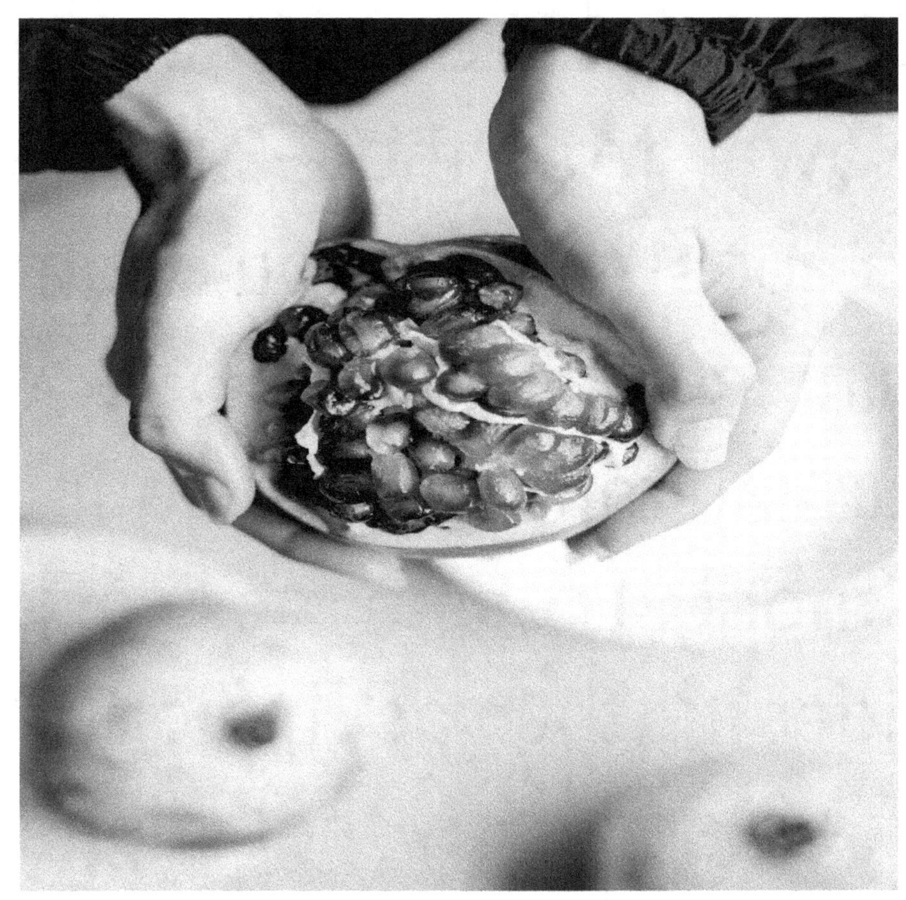

Not eating breakfast eases back
the digestion, enormous lunch and
supper feasts are an excessive lot
of food at some unacceptable

seasons of day and the body can't consume off every one of the calories.

The junk has got no other place to go than your hips and belly!

You really want to figure out how to have a moderate measured breakfast, lunch and supper with little in the middle between. Fuel the body so it consumes until you fuel it once more.

Add a lot of food to your belly and you will over fill. Try not to fuel your body and you will wear out and have no energy. Keep a predictable fuel hotspot for your body and it will end up being a consuming machine.

Learn to Balance Your Diets

A balanced diet is one that contains the six classes of food(carbohydrate, protein, vitamin, fat & oil, mineral and water).

You really want to have a reasonable plate at feasts and tidbits. What I mean is that practically every dinner needs to have a protein, carb and fat. Your body needs both protein to fix and construct slender muscle and carbs to give energy. So having a goliath bowl of pasta is certainly not a reasonable dinner however having a little part of pasta with a chicken is better.

Watch Your Weight and Maintain the Right Practices

The slight changes in weight in no less than a little while isn't sufficient to set weight reduction/gain into stone. Perseverance, over long stretches of time are the genuine proportion of progress. We are looking at ending vices that have been bringing us down for the greater part of our lives. Careless dieting is most certainly something that can destroy your weight reduction endeavors. I have seen numerous clients have their whole day demolished by the all powerful scale letting them know they are up three pounds. Quit revering the scale each day and pick one day seven days to step on the scale. Try not to let an article from your washroom floor have power in your life!

Both activity and appropriate eating should be in the image to accomplish better health and weight reduction. You can't do one and not the other. In the event that you assume you are only going to change your eating regimen and not exercise or the other way around you won't be changing your way of life. You are still in the eating routine, convenient solution mindset. Nobody said you have to go run a long distance race or at no point ever eat in the future. We are talking small steps and slow change that is "feasible" and sensible.

Eat Healthily!

Exercise Regularly!

..........and watch yourself get better, live better and look better.

Best Wishes!